HIV/TB/Diabetes Resource Kit

ZEENA NACKERDIEN

DEDICATION

To my loved ones.

DISCLAIMER

CONTENTS

ACKNOWLEDGMENTS

Thank you to all my supporters.

1 PREFACE

As outlined in the first volume, *"Perspectives on Type 2 diabetes,"* I am a South African-born US science writer with a keen interest in the escalation of Type 2 diabetes in combination with infectious diseases such as HIV/AIDS and tuberculosis in high-burden countries such as the land of my birth.

The number of resource kits for treating these diseases as independent ailments are proliferating and are available from national and international organizations. However, there seemed to be an unmet need in terms of augmenting region-specific, patient-friendly educational aids to healthcare providers that addressed the prevalence rates of HIV/AIDS, TB, and diabetes in local communities and suggested ways of overcoming some of the challenges in optimizing adherence to management of multiple ailments in one patient. While this toolkit is by no means comprehensive, the chapters are designed to provide information for the

HIV/AIDS community and a broader audience, including entrepreneurs, to use as a platform for spreading education in different languages e.g., Afrikaans, English, Ndebele, Northern Sotho, Sotho, Swazi, Tsonga, Tswana, Venda, Xhosa, and Zulu) or to supplement appropriate healthcare communications materials for their businesses with the aid of regulatory and medical organizations. Since the median age in South Africa is ≤25 years old and 30.1% of citizens were under the age of 15 according to *Wikipedia*, protecting the health of the next generation in addition to people living with HIV is of paramount importance.

Who are the groups likely to be in the frontlines of either administering or receiving treatment? Healthcare workers who play crucial roles as intermediaries between the patient and the healthcare system could benefit from an additional aid to facilitate integrated and continuous care. These workers may face the extra burden of having to deal with community- and hospital-acquired infections (HAIs) as a significant contributor to the rise in multi-drug resistant (MDR) TB in particular regions of the country. Ultimately, clinically- and legally-compliant best practices integrated into mobile clinics or other healthcare settings may contribute to improved health-related quality of life and lowering of the financial impact of treatment.

In addition, healthy, knowledgeable teachers are

one of the best defenses that children in the developing world have against the indirect impact of HIV/AIDS on negative educational outcomes. According to a recent systematic review, HIV/AIDS-orphan hood or caregiver HIV/AIDS-sickness impacted indirectly on educational outcomes via the poverty and internalizing problems that they occasioned.[3] Moreover, the HIV incidence among young women [15-24 years old] remain high relative to the rest of the population.[4] By addressing HIV/AIDS education in group settings at secondary and tertiary levels, peers and future teachers may be able to mitigate the impact of this epidemic and related illnesses

Therefore the remaining 5 chapters describe:

- Advances in HIV and TB therapies
- Disease prevalence rates in South Africa, reinvigorated national response, and treatment challenges
- Influence of comorbidities and integrated care approaches
- Based on the premise that prevention and early treatment of any disease can best be facilitated through multifaceted communication, an educational & feedback questionnaire section for patients and lay educators have been included in Chapter 5
- A supplementary table and references are

compiled in Chapter 6

2. HIV AND TB THERAPIES: THE GOOD NEWS

Given the treatment progress that has been made, the nineteen eighties, a decade that saw the HIV/AIDS health crisis bloom in the USA, seems like a blurry video from a distant past. Gone are the days of researchers haggling about the cause of a sexually transmitted infection (STI) that initially occurred in clustered outbreaks among homosexuals, hemophiliacs receiving tainted blood, and drug users. Thanks to advocacy and eventual cooperation among the different stakeholders, core realities emerged about the disease. Likewise, improved sanitation and the "golden era" of antibiotics seemed to put TB, historically known as phthisis, consumption, and "the white plague" firmly in the national rear-view mirror. Americans could be forgiven for thinking that diseases that no longer vied to replace international strife on the daily RSS feeds were now part of another era, viewable on-demand if they were consumed with a case of nostalgia.

Two factors negate the rosy view that HIV and TB are essentially cured or controlled illnesses. As outlined in my blog post, *Why HIV/AIDS should matter*, the global decrease in the disease has been offset by an increase in new HIV infections, mostly in sub-Saharan Africa and most notably in South Africa *"(between 1999 and 2008; an estimated 12.2%of South Africans were infected with the virus in 2012). Examples of other region-specific case increases are e.g., New Jersey; HIV cases diagnosed among Hispanics in Florida increased by 76% and Ugandan HIV prevalence rates rose from 6.4% in 2005/6 to 7.2% in 2012). Although the transformation of the disease into a chronic ailment is cause for celebration, HIV/AIDS remains expensive to treat (up to $402,000 discounted average lifetime costs depending on disease status). In addition, early diagnosis and effective treatment is important in order to improve quality-of-life estimates and reduce HIV transmissions. Moreover, the presence of dormant, undetectable amounts of HIV in cells may make it difficult to eradicate all vestiges of this rapidly-changing virus."*[5]

The global presence of immunocompromised or aging subpopulations with HIV/AIDS, end of the golden era when one antibiotic or the "right combination of drugs" seemed to "permanently" eradicate a pathogen, emergence of health-care associated infections (HAIs) as a threat to public safety, a proportion of healthcare professionals who may be susceptible to HAIs for various reasons, has contributed to a resurgence of "super-bugs," including multi-drug-resistant (MDR) TB.

Currently, the standard-of-care for HIV/AIDS depends on the stage of the disease. Antiretroviral therapy (ART) forms the backbone of treatment and, in some cases preventive strategies, coupled with behavioral changes for HIV⁺-individuals e.g., regular checkups, exercise, and nutritious diet, and rest. ARTs are divided into four classes depending on how they stop HIV from replicating in the body i.e., nucleoside/nucleotide reverse transcriptase inhibitors (NRTIs), non-nucleoside reverse transcriptase inhibitors (NNRTIs), protease inhibitors (PIs), and entry/fusion inhibitors.[6] According to US resources, tailored HIV therapy to control the disease is recommended if any of the following criteria applies to the patient: severe HIV symptoms, opportunistic infection. CD4 count of 350 cells/mm^3 or less, pregnancy, or HIV-related kidney disease.[7] Depending on the stage of the disease, it may take some time to determine the right combination of approved drugs and dosages for any given patient. In the meantime, patients may report short-term side effects e.g., anemia (abnormality in red blood cells), diarrhea, dizziness, fatigue, headaches, nausea and vomiting, pain and nerve problems and a rash. It is important to weigh the benefits/risks of staying on any particular regimen with a healthcare provider and immediately report long-term side-effects such as lipodystrophy, insulin resistance, lipid abnormalities, lowered bone density, and lactic acidosis.[8] However, the discovery of new drugs with new mechanisms of action offer hope that innovative combination regimens will provide the best opportunity for clinical responses and remission. As of 2014, more than 40 HIV therapies were in various stages of clinical development. One approach undergoing investigation is the modification of a patient's own genes, to make immune cells resistant to HIV and related infections. Another approach relies on therapeutic vaccination to induce a protection against viral infection. Attachment inhibitors i.e., preventing HIV from attaching and breaking through the cellular membrane, are among the different ARTs currently under evaluation.[9]

People with HIV are more likely to contract TB compared with their healthy counterparts. Recommendations to minimize the emergence of antibiotic resistance include administering a combination of rifampicin, isoniazid, pyrazinamide and ethambutol for 2 months followed by 4 months of rifampicin and isoniazid to treat active TB.[10] Nevertheless, transmission of MDR-*Mycobacterium tuberculosis* and the presence of extensively-drug resistant (XDR)-TB, sometimes in high-risk areas such as healthcare settings, are known challenges to effectively managing both diseases. The anti-TB therapy pipeline received in a boost in 2012 with the FDA-approval of the anti-TB drug in more than 40 years i.e., the diarylquinoline, bedaquiline. Six classes of chemical compounds are currently being screened for their utility as potential anti-TB drugs i.e., two nitroimidazoles (PA-824 and OPC-67683), a diarylquinoline (TMC207), an imidazopyridine amide (Q203), a diethylene diamine (SQ109), and a benzothiazinone (BTZ043). [10] As in the case of HIV, an effective TB vaccine would seem like the best treatment strategy and avoid concerns about antibiotic resistance. While the *Mycobacterium bovis* bacillus Calmette-Guerin (BCG) vaccine shows efficacy in disease prevention and progression of more severe forms of the illness in infants, the vaccine is less effective in preventing active TB in older individuals. Fourteen vaccine candidates belonging to different classes e.g., adjuvant-subunit, viral-vectored, recombinant, and whole-cell, are currently undergoing clinical evaluation.[11]

3 SOUTH AFRICA: A HIGH-BURDEN DISEASE CASE STUDY

Acquired immunodeficiency syndrome (AIDS) — a chronic immune system illness leaving an individual prone to opportunistic infections and cancers — is caused primarily by human immunodeficiency virus type 1 (HIV-1). Thus far, HIV-2 infections have mainly been found in West Africa. AIDS usually results after a 5 to 10-year incubation period in untreated HIV[+]-individuals, although a more aggressive strain of HIV has recently been reported to be associated with a faster progression to the syndrome (3 years).[12] South Africa had the highest number of new HIV infections in 2012, leads the world in terms of latent tuberculosis (TB) infections, and is vulnerable to a hidden epidemic of Type 2 diabetes that can impact the optimal management of the aforementioned infectious diseases. The national prevalence rates and related deaths attributed to these linked illnesses are indicated in (**Table 1**).[2,4,13,14]

There are differences in the proportions of new HIV infections among different provinces, implying that best practices are not reaching all affected individuals. In addition, 15-24 year-old South Africans remain disproportionately affected by new HIV infections.[4] If one believes recent estimates that the primary school completion rate is 86.4%,[11] it follows that overall improvement in general education coupled with educational aids targeted to youths and other vulnerable groups could contribute to enhancing understanding about the disease and lay the foundation for HIV[+]-individuals successfully managing the infection and other comorbidities as adults. "Catch-them-early" is a mantra that applies both to the disease and the education of patients.

Despite the statistics (**Table 1**), the South African government deserves praise for investing a significant portion of its domestic resources in a national ART rollout campaign. Life expectancy of treated individuals have been prolonged by 5 years compared with the height of the epidemic. Based on the National Strategic Plan (2012-2016) developed to address the health crisis, similar target populations with high burdens of infection have also been identified in the country e.g., men who have sex with men (MSM), women, children, sex workers, and people who inject drugs. Apart from increased counseling, home-based HIV testing and mobile clinics such as *Tutu Tester Mobile Clinics*, named in honor of anti-apartheid activist, Anglican Archbishop Desmond Tutu, have also gained in popularity in recent years. A voluntary male circumcision campaign, elevated distribution of male condoms, and the introduction of a *HIV and AIDS Life Skills Education Programme* point to a country determined to reverse the negative course of the HIV epidemic.[15] The various communication campaigns have yielded positive results among youths in terms of increased condom usage, counseling, and male circumcisions, with a concomitant decline in disease incidence in 2008-2012 compared with the pre-ART and early-ART rollout years of 2002-2005 (60% reduction in HIV incidence).[4]

Succinctly put: HIV prevention works. However, according to 2013 UNAIDS estimates, 75% of all new HIV infections occurred in sub-Saharan Africa, and the proportion of new infections in South Africa was very high (16%) compared with other countries in the region such as Zimbabwe (3%), Mozambique (5%), Kenya (5%), and Uganda (7%).[16]

While the high number of new HIV infections in South Africa (469,000)[4] may partially reflect intensified case-finding, there is no doubt that significant obstacles remain in providing lifesaving treatment to those who need it and to sustain treatment for patients already receiving care. In a resource-poor country like South Africa, there are a few glimmers of hope when it comes to improving treatment adherence with the aid of peer-peer support e.g., task-shifting and ART-adherence clubs. The former process refers to the promising approach of increasing the number of access points at which patients could receive treatment e.g., nurses (rather than doctors) initiated ART; lay counsellors (rather than nurses) carried out HIV tests; and pharmacy assistants (rather than pharmacists) prescribed ARTs.[15] Government-led processes such as nurse-initiated ART have met with promising results in primary care settings. In addition, ART-adherence clubs located in Khayelitsha (Western Cape) South Africa) focused on nurturing an atmosphere of peer support among selected HIV+-individuals and appropriate patients were recommended for intensified treatment, with the option of returning to the group under pre-specified conditions. By the end of 2012 (after adoption of the phased ART rollout by the Western Cape), more than 600 ART clubs in Khayelitsha were able to facilitate the rapid delivery of ART to

16,000 patients.[17] Evans summarized the challenges that exist with nurse-initiated management of ARTs as follows: *"Although the shift to nurse-initiated care has already begun, it does have its limitations, the main ones being adequate and sustainable training, support and salaries for staff in new roles, the integration of new members into healthcare teams, and compliance with regulatory bodies."*[18]

Add to this assessment, 2012 data showing that HIV incidence rates among women (15 to 24 years old) were over four-fold higher than among men in the same age bracket (2.5% vs. 0.6%) and that 79.2% of national survey respondents believed that they were not at risk for acquiring HIV, and the need for sustained education to maintain disease awareness becomes clear.[4] Stigma — an ongoing problem that may undermine effective messaging[19-25] and affect perceptions — can also be addressed through continuous education.

The elephant in the room is the fact that one-third of HIV+-individuals across the globe are also infected with TB. According to Evans, South Africa is no exception, ranking 4th among 22 high-burden countries.[18] The highly-desired goal of integrating largely-separate management programs is prominently featured in the National Strategic Plan,[2] as are separate perspectives on the challenges in achieving this target within the existing health system.[26]

4 IN THE SHADOW OF HIV: TB & DIABETES

TB, a potentially lethal infection caused by *M. tuberculosis*, is the leading cause of death in South Africa. [27] According to Wang et al., anti-TB treatment can cure most patients with TB, with a 2-year recurrence rate of 2% to 3%. This recurrence rate can be further lowered through directly-observed therapy (short-course, also known as DOTS).[28] DOTS remains at the heart of the *Stop TB strategy* and is comprised of 5 elements: political commitment with increased and sustained financing; case detection through quality-assured bacteriology; standardized treatment, with supervision and patient support; an effective drug supply and management system; monitoring and evaluation system, and impact measurement.[29] In an ideal world, extension of the approved regimen >6 months would eliminate extra-pulmonary, drug-resistant bacteria. Similarly, prolonging treatment is recommended when the regimen is modified because of adverse events, treatment failure, or nonadherence.[29] In addition , the alarming increase in MDR- and XDR-TB among healthcare professionals in KwaZulu Natal (2012 data; MDR-TB-related proportion of hospitalizations [per 100,000] of healthcare workers vs. non-healthcare workers: 64.8 vs. 11.9; 2012 data; XDR-TB-related proportion of hospitalizations [per 100,000] of healthcare workers vs. non-healthcare workers: 7.2 vs. 1.1),[2] highlights additional factors i.e., the contributions of HAIs or potentially susceptible healthcare professionals that have to be considered when designing a TB treatment strategy.

Compounding the optimization of TB treatment, is evidence from the literature indicating that diabetes was the most common systemic comorbidity of patients with TB, at least in Taiwan. Moreover, a separate meta-analysis indicated an increased relative risk of TB recurrence in diabetics compared with non-diabetics.[28] According to references cited by Wang et al, *"TB can worsen diabetic control through infection-related glucose intolerance or hyperglycemia caused by interactions between oral hypoglycemic drugs and anti-TB drugs, especially rifampicin."* [28] The unfavorable outcomes associated with having TB and diabetes were confirmed by the authors own studies. They suggested prolonging anti-TB treatment by 3 months in diabetics may provide the benefit of lowering recurrence rates in diabetics when treatment is not supervised.[28]

Depending on the constituents of anti-TB therapies, shorter courses of treatment have been proposed to be simpler, more cost-effective, have an acceptable safety profile and to be potentially efficacious in subsets of TB patients. Together with clinical trial results indicating that shortening anti-TB treatment did not improve clinical outcomes compared with the standard 6-month regimen,[30] the conclusions drawn by Wang et al. indicates the complexity involved in tailoring evidence-based treatment to patients in the real world.

South Africa is one of the epicenters for dealing with these two diseases in addition to HIV. Most of the world's 387 million diabetics (up to 90%) have been identified as having the Type 2 form of the disease i.e. they do not produce sufficient insulin, due to many risk factors, including a sedentary lifestyle and diet. According to Oni et al and other researchers, South Africa has one of the highest prevalence rates of Type 2 diabetes in Sub-Saharan Africa and also the highest burden of hypertension in the >50 year-old population.[31] The trend towards children who are overweight or obese[32] may lower the age at which Type 2 diabetes and associated complications have to be treated in patients with one, two or more diseases.

The coexistence of multiple infectious diseases and non-infectious co-morbidities such as diabetes within any given patient represents a treatment challenge that cannot easily be addressed in a randomized clinical trial. Currently, the closest approximation is the Population Effects of Antiretroviral Therapy to Reduce HIV Transmission (PopART) Trial [NCT01900977]. The research question being posed can be paraphrased as follows: Is a combination strategy anchored in home-based HIV testing and facilitated linkage of HIV-infected persons to care through community health workers, and universal ART therapy for seropositive persons regardless of CD4+ cell count or HIV viral load a viable way to manage HIV and STIs? Patients are currently being recruited for a clinical trial to answer this question and to further reduce the risk of HIV acquisition among uninfected individuals. The study aims to expand voluntary medical male circumcision, diagnosis and treatment of STIs, behavioral counseling, and condom distribution. In addition, the study also incorporates promotion of other interventions designed to reduce HIV and TB transmission, including optimization of the prevention of mother-to-child HIV transmission and enhanced individual and public health TB services.

Perhaps results from this trial would provide a foundation for best practices for the integrated care of infectious diseases that can then be combined with real-world management of diabetes. This will become necessary as more and more successfully-treated, HIV$^+$-individuals will likely live longer and hence have an increased risk of acquiring a non-communicable disease such as Type 2 diabetes.

5 EDUCATION

The profound impact of co-infections and non-infectious illnesses on exacerbating HIV/AIDS and TB has garnered global attention and different frameworks are being funded to address region-specific interventions. It is beyond the scope of this resource guide to delve into each program. In the absence of large-scale, expanded, optimal integrated care operating within functional health systems, this chapter will focus on prevention and early recognition of symptoms of the three illnesses under discussion. Together with information from official sources geared towards empowering patients, the aim of this chapter is to facilitate affected individuals' abilities to understand and exercise control over the management of their illnesses or better yet, to be vigilant in preventing the onset of HIV/AIDS, TB, and diabetes. Recorded health information should in all cases be evaluated in cooperation with a healthcare professional.

Prevention/management of HIV/AIDS

Risk factors[33]

Anyone regardless of race, religion, gender, age (even unborn children can get the disease) or sexual orientation is at risk of contracting HIV. The risk increases if one has multiple sexual partners.

Key risk factors are:

- Having unprotected sex
- Having another STI
- Being an uncircumcised man
- Using intravenous drugs

Vulnerable populations include men who have sex with men, transgender persons, people who inject drugs, sex workers and their clients, and HIV--individuals in relationships with HIV+-individuals or those at higher risk of exposure to HIV. Specific migrant groups are also at heightened risk of HIV exposure. [2]

Symptoms[34]

Symptoms alone are not indicative of the disease. The only way to know for sure if you have HIV is to get tested.

- During the latency stage (on average 10 years, but some people may progress faster to the symptomatic stage), HIV+- individuals may be asymptomatic or exhibit mild symptoms. A person can transmit the virus even at this early stage of the disease
- A constellation of clinical symptoms (e.g.,

fever, swollen glands, sore throat, rash, fatigue, muscle and joint aches and pains, headache) lasting up to a few weeks may suggest a need for initial rapid point-of-care diagnosis with e.g. the US FDA-approved *Alere Determine™ HIV-1/2 Ag/Ab Combo* test and HIV-serostatus confirmation with laboratory diagnostic evaluation (US Centers for Disease Control and Prevention, 2014: Laboratory Testing for HIV Infection, Updated Recommendations)[35]

- During the late stages of untreated HIV, patients may exhibit the following symptoms: rapid weight loss, recurring fever or profuse night sweats, extreme and unexplained tiredness, prolonged swelling of the lymph glands (in the armpits, groin, or neck), diarrhea that lasts for more than a week, sores (mouth, anus, or genitals), pneumonia, blotches (on or under the skin or inside the mouth, nose, or eyelids), memory loss, depression, and other neurologic disorders

Prevention tips[34]

- Being aware of a sex partner's HIV serostatus (results from any home-based diagnostic kit should be verified by a follow-up visit to the doctor) is an important first step. Monogamy or delayed sexual debut alone cannot prevent HIV/AIDS, as the infectious disease can be transmitted by a spouse or long-term partner

o Although ART can prolong life once someone has HIV and post-exposure prophylaxis (taking anti-HIV medications as soon as possible after exposure to the virus)[36] may reduce the chance of becoming HIV[+], it is still important to use condoms during sex

o Proper use of a condoms[37] will reduce the risk of transmission via vaginal, oral or anal sex

- Researchers are working on microbicides as an alternative for people who do not wish to use condoms or who are unable to resist coercion to have unprotected sex. However, currently there is no effective microbicide or vaccine that can prevent HIV infection

- In addition to male condoms, female condoms could be an alternative for women to use as contraception and to reduce the risk of HIV infection or another STI. The Universal Access to Female Condoms (UAFC) Joint Program has two country-wide projects in Nigeria and Cameroon.

> In addition, UAFC condoms went on sale in South Africa in 2013

- Intravenous drug users should use sterile equipment and water and never share equipment with others.
  - o Although HIV is primarily spread through sex, one can also contract the disease through sharing needles

Prevention/management of pulmonary TB
Risk factors[38]

- Birth in an endemic country
- HIV infection
- Diabetes
- Immunosuppressive medications
- Exposure to infection
- Silicosis (a disease caused by inhaling silica dust)
- Apical fibrosis (scarring of specific lung lobe regions)

Vulnerable populations: include household contacts of confirmed TB cases, including infants and young children; healthcare workers, mine workers, correctional services staff and inmates; children and adults living with HIV; diabetics and people who are malnourished; smokers, drug users and alcohol abusers; mobile, migrant and refugee populations; people living and working in poorly ventilated and overcrowded environments, including those who live in informal settlements.[2]

Symptoms[38]

Screening of high-risk populations (by trained professionals) is recommended in endemic countries as a first step to control the disease

- Common symptoms include fever, cough, anorexia, weight loss, malaise, and night sweats (consult a doctor for a complete medical examination)

Prevention tips[39]

- Keep your germs to yourself if you have active TB. It usually takes a few weeks of treatment with appropriate medications before you are not contagious to friends and family. The following tips may be helpful:
  - Stay home during the first few weeks of active TB
  - Open up your windows, ventilate the room, and use a fan to blow indoor air outside (providing it is not winter). TB spreads easier in enclosed spaces
  - Cover your mouth every time you laugh, sneeze, or cough (used tissues should be discarded in a sealed bag)
  - Wearing a surgical mask during the first three weeks of active TB may lessen the risk of transmission
- Complete your entire course of treatment as per medical instructions

o Remember to inform your doctor/nurse of any non-TB medications or over-the-counter drugs. The possibility exists that some of these drugs may lessen the efficacy of TB-specific treatment

- In TB-endemic countries, the BCG vaccine is available to prevent severe TB in children.
    o However, it is not recommended for general use as it is not very effective in adults. Alternative vaccine options are still being evaluated in clinical trials

Prevention/management of Type 2 diabetes[40]

Risk factors

The South African Medical Research Council reports that 61% of the population is overweight, obese, or severely obese,[41] and many of these individuals are likely to be youths.

Factors that predispose youths to diabetes are: [40]

- Being overweight or a lack of exercise
- Race: The Indian population in South Africa has a strong genetic predisposition (11-13%), followed by coloreds (8-10%), blacks (5-8%), and whites (4%)[42]
- Family history of Type 2 diabetes
- Having been exposed to gestational diabetes prior to birth
- One or more conditions in organs other than the pancreas such as increased fatty deposits in the liver, patchy skin discoloration (on the

neck and under the arms) known as *acanthosis nigricans*, and a condition in women that include no menstrual periods, unusual hair growth and being overweight (polycystic ovarian syndrome)

- High blood pressure or levels of fat/cholesterol in blood can be a risk factor and also contribute to complications associated with the disease

Taking certain medications for mental health conditions (consult with a healthcare provider)

Vulnerable populations include those whose who are overweight, follow an unhealthy diet, are physically inactive, have high blood pressure/gestational diabetes/family history of the disease, belong to certain ethnic groups, or have an impaired glucose tolerance test (guideline-defined pre-diabetes, otherwise known as higher than normal blood glucose that falls below the threshold for diagnosing diabetes).[1]

Symptoms

Children may be asymptomatic and only diagnosed when visiting the doctor for other reasons e.g., being overweight.

Clinical symptoms include:[40]

- Being tired
- Yeast infections
- Blurred vision
- Increase in feeling thirsty
- Going to the bathroom more

Prevention tips[40]

Parents should, where possible, adopt a healthy eating and lifestyle example for children. Suggested lifestyle changes to consider are:

- Opt for water instead of sugary drinks
- Fresh fruits and cut-up veggies are healthy alternatives to processed snacks
- Get moving. Children should get at least 60 minutes of exercise daily.
- Replace excessive sedentary activities such as watching TV for more than 2 hours at a stretch with activity play time.
- Follow nutritional guides under the guidance of a healthcare provider

Sample questionnaires

Rather than being prescriptive, the sample questionnaires are intended to serve as suggestions for educators and activists on quick quizzes to poll student knowledge and to solicit feedback from pre-teens, teenagers and young adults, and educators. Sources used to compile the sample surveys and this document contain the answers and can serve as study materials. Users of this guide may wish to generate online forms or, in the absence of computers or access to social media, prepare hand-written materials.

HIV/AIDS questionnaire[43,44]

* Required

1. Do all people with HIV have AIDS? *

     [ ] Yes

     [ ] No

2. Can I get AIDS from sharing a cup or shaking hands with someone who has HIV or AIDS? *

     [ ] Yes

     [ ] No

3. Can HIV be transmitted through an insect bite? *

     [ ] Yes

     [ ] No

4. Can I get HIV from kissing? *

     [ ] Yes

     [ ] No

5. Does abstinence include anal sex? *

  [ ] Yes

  [ ] No

6. How effective are latex condoms in preventing **HIV**? Rating scale starts from **1** (not very effective) to **5** (extremely effective)

  1 2 3 4 5

7. If you had sex the previous night with someone that you suspect has **HIV** and the condom broke during the act, what should be done? *

a. What are the next steps when you are diagnosed with **HIV**? *

b. Why do you think it is/is not important to teach students about **HIV/AIDS**? *

8. How do you feel the course should be presented in order to make people comfortable with the topic? *

TB questionnaire [45]

* Required

1. What is TB and what are the risk factors for the disease? *

2. What is latent TB and how does it differ from active TB? *

3. How is TB spread? *

4. Should everyone get tested for TB? *

5. What if an individual has an HIV infection? *

6. How is drug-sensitive TB treated in the developing world? *

What are the serious side effects of the most common TB medications? *

What is multidrug-resistant and extensively-drug resistant TB?

How can one keep from spreading TB? *

What do you feel needs to be done to improve TB management among vulnerable groups? *

Diabetes questionnaire [46]

* Required

What is Type 2 diabetes? *

Name all the symptoms suggesting a need to be tested for the disease. *

Name at least three risk factors for Type 2 diabetes. *

How is Type 2 diabetes treated? *

Can patient education be improved? If so, how? *

6 APPENDIX

Table 1: Estimated HIV/AIDS, TB and diabetes profiles for South Africa (2008-2014 data) [2,4,13,14]

Disease (Year)	People living with profiled diseases	National prevalence (%)	Deaths
HIV (2012 data)	6.4 million	12.2	
TB (2012 data, new infections; 2008-2011 mortalities)	~400,000[†]	n.a.	54,112
HIV/TB (2011 data)	211,800 (65% of screened patients)	n.a.	
Diabetes (2014 data)[a]	2,713.4[b]	8.4	68,977[c]

[a]Diagnosed Type 1 and 2 diabetics (20-79 years old); [b]Number of diabetics (estimated in thousands); [c]Overall number of estimated diabetes-related deaths (20-79 years old); [†]1.8% of all new cases had multi-drug resistant TB; n.a., not available; Globally, there were 35 million people living with HIV and 9 million new TB cases identified at the end of 2013.[47,48]. Approximately 10.6% of South Africans are living with HIV.[4] This translates into an estimated 6.4 million people living with HIV — by far the largest number people in one country living with this pathogen and second-only to Swaziland (27.4%) in terms of global HIV prevalence.[4,47] HIV can weaken the immune system, leaving individuals prone to sexually transmitted infections (STIs) or prone to developing other illnesses caused by opportunistic pathogens such as TB – currently the leading cause of death in South Africa.[27] A hidden epidemic of diabetes has, in turn, been associated with increased TB.[49] Overall, worldwide access to ARTs has had a profound effect on reducing HIV-related deaths, including South Africa (an estimated decline of HIV-related deaths from 410,000 in 2010 to 200,000 in 2013).[50]

References

1. International Diabetes Federation. Risk Factors. 2014.

2. South African National Aids Council. Progress report on the National Strategic plan for HIV, TB, and STIs (2012 - 2016) 2014; http://www.sanac.org.za/publications/reports/cat_view/7-publications/9-reports.

3. Orkin M, Boyes ME, Cluver LD, Zhang Y. Pathways to poor educational outcomes for HIV/AIDS-affected youth in South Africa. *AIDS Care.* 2013;26(3):343-350.

4. Human Sciences Research Council. South African National HIV Prevalence, Incidence and Behaviour Survey, 2012. 2014; http://www.hsrc.ac.za/uploads/pageContent/4565/SABSSM%20IV%20LEO%20final.pdf. Accessed May, 2014.

5. Nackerdien Z. Why HIV/AIDS should matter. Norwalk Patch.

6. U.S. Department of Health and Human Services (AIDSInfo) Overview for HIV treatments. 2014; https://www.aids.gov/hiv-aids-basics/just-diagnosed-with-hiv-aids/treatment-options/overview-of-hiv-treatments/. Accessed March, 2015.

7. U.S. Department of Health and Human Services (AIDSInfo) Reasons to start

treatment. 2014; https://www.aids.gov/hiv-aids-basics/just-diagnosed-with-hiv-aids/treatment-options/reasons-to-start-treatment/index.html. Accessed March, 2015.

8. U.S. Department of Health and Human Services (AIDSInfo) What are side effects? 2014; https://www.aids.gov/hiv-aids-basics/just-diagnosed-with-hiv-aids/treatment-options/side-effects/index.html. Accessed March, 2015.

9. Pharmaceutical and Manufacturing Researchers Association. Medicines in development for HIV/AIDS. Biopharmaceutical Company Researchers Are Developing More Than 40 Medicines and Vaccines For HIV Infection Treatment and Prevention. 2014; http://www.phrma.org/sites/default/files/pdf/2014-meds-in-dev-hiv-aids.pdf. Accessed April, 2015.

10. Lechartier B, Rybniker J, Zumla A, Cole ST. *Tuberculosis drug discovery in the post-post-genomic era.* 2014.

11. da Costa C, Walker B, Bonavia A. Tuberculosis Vaccines - state of the art, and novel approaches to vaccine development. *Int J Infect Dis.* 2015;32:5-12.

12. Kouri V, Khouri R, Alemán Y, et al. CRF19_cpx is an Evolutionary fit HIV-1

Variant Strongly Associated With Rapid Progression to AIDS in Cuba. *EBioMedicine.* 2015.

13. International Diabetes Federation. IDF Diabetes Atlas, 6th edn. Brussels, Belgium: International Diabetes Federation. 2014; http://www.idf.org/diabetesatlas. Accessed May, 2014.

14. TB Facts.org. Information about tuberculosis. TB in South Africa - National and Provincial Statistics. Headline TB Statistics for South Africa. 2015; http://www.tbfacts.org/tb-statistics-south-africa.html. Accessed March, 2015.

15. AVERT (Averting HIV and AIDS). HIV and AIDS in South Africa. 2014; http://www.avert.org/hiv-aids-south-africa.htm.

16. UNAIDS. The Gap Report. 2014; http://www.unaids.org/sites/default/files/en/media/unaids/contentassets/documents/unaidspublication/2014/UNAIDS_Gap_report_en.pdf. Accessed April, 2015.

17. Wilkinson LS. ART adherence clubs: A long-term retention strategy for clinically stable patients receiving antiretroviral therapy. *South African Journal of HIV Medicine.* 2013;14(2).

18. Evans D. Ten years on ART – where to now? *SAMJ.* 2013;103(4).

19. Link B, Phelan J. Stigma and its public health implications. *Lancet.* 2006;367(9509):528 - 529.
20. Stangl A, Grossman C. Global action to reduce HIV stigma and discrimination. *J Int AIDS Soc.* 2012;16:2.
21. dos Santos M, Kruger P, Mellors S, Wolvaardt G, van der Ryst E. An exploratory survey measuring stigma and discrimination experienced by people living with HIV/AIDS in South Africa: the People Living with HIV Stigma Index. *BMC Public Health.* 2014;14(1):80.
22. Magadzire BP, Budden A, Ward K, Jeffery R, Sanders D. Frontline health workers as brokers: provider perceptions, experiences and mitigating strategies to improve access to essential medicines in South Africa. *BMC Health Services Research.* 2014;14:520.
23. Valdiserri R. HIV/AIDS stigma: an impediment to public health. *Am J Public Health.* 2012;92(3):341 - 342.
24. Brown L, Macintyre K. Interventions to reduce HIV/AIDS stigma: What have we learned? *AIDS Educ Prev.* 2003;15(1):49 - 69.
25. Kalichman S, Simbayi L. Traditional beliefs about the cause of AIDS and AIDS-related stigma in South Africa. *AIDS Care.* 2004;16(5):572 - 580.

26. Coovadia H, Jewkes R, Barron P, Sanders D, McIntyre D. The health and health system of South Africa: historical roots of current public health challenges. *The Lancet.*374(9692):817-834.

27. Department of Health. South Africa. Joint Review of HIV, TB, and PTMCT programmes in South Africa. 2013; http://www.health.gov.za/. Accessed March, 2015.

28. Wang J-Y, Lee M-C, Shu C-C, et al. Optimal duration of anti-tb treatment in patients with diabetes: Nine or six months? *Chest.* 2015;147(2):520-528.

29. World Health Organization. The five elements of DOTS. 2015; http://www.who.int/tb/dots/whatisdots/en/.

30. Merle CS, Fielding K, Sow OB, et al. A Four-Month Gatifloxacin-Containing Regimen for Treating Tuberculosis. *New England Journal of Medicine.* 2014;371(17):1588-1598.

31. Oni T, Youngblood E, Boulle A, McGrath N, Wilkinson RJ, Levitt NS. Patterns of HIV, TB, and non-communicable disease multi-morbidity in peri-urban South Africa- a cross sectional study. *BMC Infect Dis.* 2015;15(1):20.

32. Armstrong ME, Lambert MI, Lambert EV. Secular trends in the prevalence of stunting,

overweight and obesity among South African children (1994-2004). *Eur J Clin Nutr.* 2011;65(7):835-840.

33. Mayo Clinic. Diseases and Conditions a: HIV/AIDS Risk factors. 2014; http://www.mayoclinic.org/diseases-conditions/hiv-aids/basics/risk-factors/con-20013732. Accessed March, 2015.

34. U.S. Department of Health and Human Services (AIDSInfo)b. Offering information about HIV/AIDS Treatment, Prevention, and Research) Prevention. HIV/AIDS 101. Signs and Symptoms. 2014; https://www.aids.gov/hiv-aids-basics/hiv-aids-101/signs-and-symptoms/. Accessed March, 2015.

35. US Centers for Disease Control and Prevention. Laboratory Testing for Diagnosis of HIV Infection (Updated). 2014; http://www.cdc.gov/hiv/pdf/HIVtestingAlgorithmRecommendation-Final.pdf.

36. U.S. Department of Health and Human Services (AIDSInfo)d. Post-exposure prophylaxis. 2014; https://www.aids.gov/frequently-asked-questions/. Accessed March, 2015.

37. The Nemours Foundation. TeensHealth. Condom. 1995-2015; http://kidshealth.org/teen/sexual_health/co

ntraception/contraception_condom.html. Accessed March, 2015.

38. Epocrates (An Athena Health Company) online: Pulmonary Tuberculosis. 2015; https://online.epocrates.com/u/2944165/Pulmonary+tuberculosis. Accessed March, 2015.

39. Mayo Clinic. Diseases and Conditions b: Tuberculosis. Prevention. . 2014; http://www.mayoclinic.org/diseases-conditions/tuberculosis/basics/prevention/con-20021761. Accessed March, 2015.

40. Canadian Diabetes Association. Children and Type 2 diabetes. 2015; http://www.diabetes.ca/diabetes-and-you/kids-teens-diabetes/children-type-2-diabetes. Accessed March, 2015.

41. Baleta A, Mitchell F. Country in Focus: diabetes and obesity in South Africa. *The Lancet Diabetes & Endocrinology.* 2014;2(9):687-688.

42. health24. Diabetes: Prevalence of diabetes in South Africa. 2014; http://www.health24.com/Medical/Diabetes/About-diabetes/Diabetes-tsunami-hits-South-Africa-20130210. Accessed March, 2015.

43. Wood L, Rens J. Treating 'AIDS blindness': A critical pedagogical approach to HIV

education at tertiary level. *African Journal of AIDS Research.* 2014;13(1):65-73.

44. U.S. Department of Health and Human Services (AIDSInfo)c. Offering information about HIV/AIDS Treatment, Prevention, and Research) Frequently asked questions. 2014; https://www.aids.gov/frequently-asked-questions/. Accessed March, 2015.

45. United States Centers for Disease Control and Prevention. Questions and answers about TB. 2014; http://www.cdc.gov/tb/publications/faqs/.

46. Hess-Fischl A. endocrineweb. Type 2 Diabetes FAQ. 1997-2015; http://www.endocrineweb.com/conditions/type-2-diabetes/type-2-diabetes-faq.

47. Henry J. Kaiser Family Foundation. The Global HIV/AIDS Epidemic. 2014; http://kff.org/global-health-policy/fact-sheet/the-global-hivaids-epidemic/. Accessed March, 2015.

48. World Health Organization. Global Tuberculosis Report. 2014; http://apps.who.int/iris/bitstream/10665/137094/1/9789241564809_eng.pdf. Accessed February, 2015.

49. Ronacher K, Joosten SA, van Crevel R, Dockrell HM, Walzl G, Ottenhoff TH. Acquired immunodeficiencies and

tuberculosis: focus on HIV/AIDS and diabetes mellitus. *Immunol Rev.* 2015;264(1):121-137.

50. Mee P, Collinson MA, Madhavan S, et al. Determinants of the risk of dying of HIV/AIDS in a rural South African community over the period of the decentralised roll-out of antiretroviral therapy: a longitudinal study. *Glob Health Action.* 2014;7:24826.

7. ABOUT THE AUTHOR

Zeena Nackerdien is a dual US and South African citizen. She obtained a PhD degree in Biochemistry from the University of Stellenbosch in South Africa. Zeena has been a research chemist at the National Institute of Standards and Technology in Maryland and a senior research associate at The Rockefeller University in New York. She is the author of several publications in scientific journals, a book chapter, a novel, and a collection of poetry. As a scientist turned patient advocate and writer, she is intensely interested in building relationships with people from different cultures through story-telling and education. Zeena currently lives in Brooklyn, New York.